Essential Oils

A Beginners Guide to Nature's Therapy

Andrea Gray *Copyright* © **2015**

Disclaimer

his or her own actions when it comes to reading the book.

Adherence to all applicable laws and regulations, including international, federal, state, and local governing professional licensing, business practices, advertising, and all other aspects of doing business in the US, Canada, or any other jurisdiction is the sole responsibility of the purchaser or reader.

Neither the author nor the publisher assumes any responsibility or liability whatsoever on the behalf of the purchaser or reader of these materials.

Any received slight of any individual or organization is purely unintentional.

Introduction

As hype over essential oils grows, and their popularity spreads, so do a lot of false claims and conflicting information causing more questions than answers, leading to a lot of confusion for beginners. What company do I trust? Do I have to dilute them? Are they really safe for my kids? Why does one say to ingest, another says not to?

Take a look at these four statements and answer true or false:

1) Since pure essential oils are natural, they are all safe to use.

2) An essential oil that is 100% pure is an excellent quality oil.

3) An aromatherapist can recommend and sell you an oil, specifically with intention of preventing, treating, or curing an illness.

4) Ingesting essential oils is always safe as long as the oils are 100% pure.

If you answered true to any these, or if you just don't know, this book is for you.

I must tell you that it's *not* a book about each oil and what you can use them for, nor is it a book of recipes. There are plenty of those to go around. As the title says, it's about understanding essential oils: what they are, how they are obtained, how they are regulated, what to consider in a company before you buy, and general safety information and precautions. I hope you find it very helpful as you journey into the fragrant world of essential oils.

Chapter 1: What Are Essential Oils

Essential oils are the foundation of a complimentary or alternative form of medicine called aromatherapy. They are highly aromatic oils obtained from various plant elements in nature, including seeds, bark, leaves, stems, flowers and more. There are thousands of different species on this Earth, but only a fraction of plants make enough oil (or any at all) and are strong enough to withstand any processes for us to obtain them. Some essential oils come from plants that are rare, or only grow in certain conditions and can be harder to obtain (for instance, sandalwood.) Others, such as those from citrus fruits like lemon, orange and grapefruit, can be much more easily accessed.

Essential oils are volatile (can evaporate), which allows us to separate them from plant matter. They aren't exactly "oil" in the way you may expect. They are lightweight, not greasy, and many have a watery feel to them even though they are not water soluble;

they will float on top of water and only mix with the aid of a solvent.

It can take several pounds or even hundreds of pounds to obtain a significant amount of oil, and by time an essential oil has been bottled for purchase it is in a highly concentrated form. Every drop contains medicinal and therapeutic properties, including (but not limited to) antiseptic, antibiotic, anti-inflammatory, and anti-fungal, and can be used as mood enhancers, aphrodisiacs, deodorants, cleansers and more. These properties can often be beneficial just by inhaling the aromas (although as you begin to experiment with various oils you will find not all have a scent you find appealing.)

You may have never purchased a bottle of essential oil, and yet used them many times already. Many oils have properties excellent for skin and hair and are found in a variety of cosmetics, perfumes, lotions, soaps, toothpaste, natural bug sprays and hair products. Several essential oils are also approved as safe for use as a food additive (GRAS – Generally regarding as safe) by the FDA, and can add a burst of flavor to a meal when used in proper amounts. They can also be used around the home for cleaning, freshening, and as bug and rodent repellents. A very popular recipe passed around social media for homemade play dough included small amounts of peppermint essential oil. Lemon essential oil is a powerful grease fighter when combined with baking soda and peroxide, and is also used as tarnish remover.

The use of essential oils in the U.S. really began in the latter decades of the 20th century, but have gained quite a bit of popularity in more recent years. They are also used in France, England, China, Germany, the Philippines, and other countries around the world.

Tip: For those who want to further their education on clinical research, I highly recommend a textbook by essential oil experts Robert Tisserand and Rodney Young: Second Edition, Essential Oil Safety. (I am in no way affiliated with them, or their book, nor have they been asked to endorse this one or promote it in anyway. This is simply a recommendation, as it's considered by many to be the most authoritative and current book on research and safety.)

Tip: There is an extensive amount of studies available for free on the governmental search engine, Pubmed. (When reviewing any studies online, remember they are an excellent source and learning tool, but must be interpreted with perspective and caution; not all are always considered reliable, some may use humans, others may use rodents or other animals for testing, plus there are any number of other factors that could influence the outcome of the results.)

The History of Essential Oils

Aromatherapy, although not given its name until the 20th century, is one of the oldest forms of medicinal practice that is still being used today. Aromas of plant matter were obtained in a variety of different ways, for various reasons, dating back to 5500 B.C. This included primitive forms of distillation, or heating plant matter over hot coals and breathing the aromas.

Essential oils in the form we know them may date back to a medieval time when alchemists were searching for a fifth element. This missing fifth element, "the quintessential" fifth element, was based on Aristotle's theory that all matter is composed of earth, air, wind and fire. The missing element was not of material substance but instead was a life force or spirit. When it was discovered that distilling plant matter would turn the aromas into vapors, they believed the vapors to be the quintessential element. Quintessential was later shortened to just essential.

Steam Distillation

The alchemists were using steam distillation, which is still the most common method for obtaining essential oils today. The desired oil's plant matter (leaves, flowers, etc.) is put into a container and then steamed. The steam causes the oils to release from the matter in the form of vapors. In a separate container the vapors are then cooled and return to their natural state of oil, along with the water from the steam. The oil is then separated from the water.

This remaining water, the byproduct of steam distillation, is known as hydrosol.

Cold Pressing

Cold Pressing, also referred to as expression, can be used on a variety of different materials, and is the purest way to obtain fixed oils/vegetable oils. With essential oils it is the common method for use on citrus fruits such as lemon, bergamot and lime. Although these fruits can be steam distilled, the heat can be disruptive or destroy the acids and chemical makeup, producing a less than desired aroma. Therefore, the peels and rinds undergo a process where the oils are punctured and released, or pressed out. Other material from the peels is released as well, so the oils are then separated.

Citrus oils that are cold pressed are phototoxic when used on the skin, and thus it's important to know the method of extraction used when buying and using them. (Citrus oils and phototoxicity will be discussed further in a later chapter.)

Steam distillation and cold pressing are considered by many to be the only way to obtain a pure essential oil; a "quintessential" oil.

Cure All

Essential Oils do not cure everything. Yes, I actually feel compelled to write that because, believe it or not, it's a growing misconception.

Just three days ago, as I was working on my final draft for this eBook, I got a call from a friend, Sarah. Her son is 7 years old and he suffers from a kidney disease. His daily life typically involves steroids and other medications, and as any parent would, she's seeking out anything that can help him. A friend of hers told her juniper berry essential oil could treat his condition, and she would happily sell her a bottle.

Sarah knows I love to promote using essential oils to anyone who will listen, but I don't sell them. She trusted me to be honest with her about the recommendation and simply asked, was this true? She probably got a little more of an answer than she bargained for, including aggravation with her friend for even suggesting such a thing. Her friend is not trained in aromatherapy, has no medical background, and clearly isn't qualified to treat a 7 year old's very life changing disease with any substance, natural or otherwise. And there is no sound evidence I can find anywhere to support the notion that this oil could help him at all (in fact, at one point in time, it was advised that those who have kidney disease should avoid it.)

This is similar to what happened to me when I was first introduced to them. Merely a week after attending a party where I learned about these miracles in a bottle, how they would completely replace all of the prescription drugs in our cabinets and fix every ailment known to mankind, my favorite Aunt in the world was told she may have leukemia. This sent me on a mission to find the oils that would cure her. My efforts led me beyond the sales people, to aromatherapists who gave me some very kind, but firm responses: there is no oil in the world proven to cure leukemia. But, wait... that's not what they said! Was I really that gullible? Maybe those who suggest they are nothing but snake oils are right. Or are they?

The fact is, there are many scientifically proven benefits to essential oils. For example, research confirms that lavender can aid with anxiety, and rosemary can improve memory. It's also proven that oils have anti-bacterial and anti-fungal properties as well, and could *possibly* be a safer alternative to certain antibiotics. And yes, they are even being studied more and more every day for *potential* capabilities in treating a variety of serious diseases, *including* cancer. But, again, they don't cure everything.

Chapter 2: Quality Vs Purity

It's very common to hear that oils from any certain company are the best because they are 100% Pure. But it's important to note that there is no official governing body to ensure the accuracy of such a claim, and even an oil that is 100% pure isn't guaranteed to be a *quality* oil.

Purity

There are a couple of factors that help determine if an oil is "pure." First, how it was obtained, and second, if it was adulterated.

As mentioned in chapter 1, only oils acquired through steam distillation or cold pressing are considered (by most) to be a true essential oil. If a solvent is used to extract the oil, it is no longer pure. (There are some oils used in aromatherapy that can *only* be obtained through solvent extraction. These will be reviewed in the next chapter.)

Adulterated, in simple terms, means another ingredient has been added to the essential oil. For example, a company could be aware that an oil is lacking in quality and therefore add synthetic ingredients. Or, they may try to cut costs and mix it with a different oil (usually cheaper) with similar chemical components.

Another form of adulteration is mixing an essential oil with a carrier oil. There are valid reasons to do this, and many companies will sell diluted oils, however when they do so without informing their consumers, it is deceitful.

Quality

There are several different factors that go into producing *quality* oils. First, is it pure. Second, the native soil, climate and temperature of where the plants are grown can cause variations in the chemistry and aromas of oils. The specific plant matter used can also affect the outcome of the oil, for example, using a plant's flowers instead of the leaves could lead to different properties and efficacy.

Quality can also be impacted by distillation. Some water soluble components *are* lost in distillation. It can't be avoided, and the fragrance of an essential oil can be somewhat different than the fragrance of its actual plant for this reason. However, many of the desired properties of the oil are preserved if proper distillation techniques are used. Likewise, if factors such as time, temperature and pressure are wrong, it can change or possibly destroy components of the oil. Nonetheless it could still be sold as a 100% pure oil.

Testing

It is possible for aromatherapists, experts, and even familiar consumers to determine just by aroma, color, or consistency if there is a problem with an oil. (Consumers will also often identify when their oil has reached its shelf life based on the altered odor.)

Once an oil passes the sniff test, a common method for testing them is typically a Gas Chromatography/Mass Spectrometry (GC/MS). Because of the sophistication of synthetic ingredients, other further analysis may be done as well. Although GC/MS and other testing can be expensive, it's important that batches of oil from suppliers are tested on a regular basis for quality and purity. These tests can show even the smallest hints of solvents and/or adulteration.

Chapter 3: Absolutes, Co2's, and Hydrosols

There are some flowers and plants that are too delicate to undergo steam distillation and need to be extracted with solvents. Although these fit loosely in the category of essential oils, these types of oils should always be properly identified, labeled and marketed.

Absolutes

Absolutes are made by a process where certain compounds are separated by an organic solvent. This forms a wax type substance called concrete. Ethanol (alcohol) or another solvent is then used to extract the fragrances from the concrete. After the ethanol evaporates, the oil is left behind. Some wax is often extracted along with the oil and can render a much thicker product than essential oils.

Because of the solvent/alcohol extraction, absolutes aren't always a popular choice for many aromatherapists. The two more commonly used absolutes are jasmine and rose. Although rose essential oil is attainable, it is very expensive due to the amount of flowers it takes to acquire it. Rose absolute is a more affordable alternative.

Solvent extraction doesn't destroy some of the aromatic compounds that steam does, and often absolutes can carry additional therapeutic properties and be more fragrant than essential oils. Due to their potency, and the possibility of containing remnants of alcohol, they are often not recommended for topical use, never recommended for ingestion, and additional precautions may be needed for use with children, or women who are pregnant.

Enfleurage

This is an ancient method that involves using fat to absorb the scents of flower petals. It is very time consuming and labor intensive and is rare and very costly. The most common enfleurage on the market is Jasmine.

A pure, lily essential oil cannot be obtained through distillation, but there are lily absolutes, and it is possible however to find a high dollar, excellent quality lily enfleurage.

CO2's

Co2's are extracted using carbon dioxide as a solvent. The process is similar to steam distilling except carbon dioxide is used in place of steam, which also eliminates the need for high heat. Even though carbon dioxide is in gas form (we exhale CO_2 from our bodies), for the distillations it is forced into a liquid state. Once the distillation is complete, the CO_2 turns back into a gas, leaving only extracts of the oil and plant material/waxes behind. How much of the plant material extracted would depend on various factors during the distillation.

CO_2 extractions result in the closest possible scent of the original source you can get, and because high heat is not required, they can have different properties, or retain more of the chemical constituents found in the actual plant. For these reasons they can be a preferred choice over essential oils, except they are much more costly to produce and thus more expensive to purchase.

For matter that is unable to be steam distilled or cold pressed, CO_2's are a favorable alternative to absolutes. In the past, Vanilla has only been available in absolute form, but with the use of carbon dioxide, a Vanilla that more closely resembles an essential oil is now able to be produced. A great benefit to using carbon dioxide is that it takes less plant matter, making it a better method for rare or harder to obtain species.

Hydrosols

Hydrosol, as previously mentioned, is the remaining water after steam distillation is complete and the oil is removed. This fragrant water still contains all of the essence of the plant, but is much less potent and a far gentler alternative to a highly concentrated oil. There are very few safety concerns with a quality hydrosol, and no dilution is necessary for topical use. They are recommended instead of essential oils for infants and children. Hydrosols can also be called hydrolats or floral waters, but not all products sold as floral waters are actual hydrosols.

Quality, freshness and storage are extremely important because unlike essential oils, hydrosols can grow bacteria very quickly. Always check with the supplier for purity of a hydrosol, as sometimes alcohol can be added as a preservative. Many vendors may ship hydrosols in plastic bottles, but they should be transferred to clear, sterile glass containers if possible.

Tips: When purchasing a large bottle of a hydrosol, rather than exposing the entire bottle to oxygen each time you need it, separate into small bottles for storage. The stored bottles should be full, leaving as little free room as possible to reduce oxygen exposure. Refrigeration is best for storage, or cool, dark places. These tips will apply to essential oils as well.

Although dark, amber bottles would be better to restrict light, clear glass containers allow for you to watch for signs of bacteria, which will manifest toward the bottom of the bottle.

Chapter 3: Chemical Compounds, Latin Names and Chemotypes

Chemical Compounds

The first time I learned about essential oils I remember asking what would work for a certain ailment. The very kind saleswoman opened a book and found it, and showed me the list of oils that could be helpful. It was overwhelming, as it felt like half of the different oils were listed. In fact, nearly every ailment in her book had so many different options. Honestly, it was confusing and I didn't even know where to start.

The fact is, many essential oils can and do have many similarities. The full scientific explanation goes well beyond this beginner's guide, but basically, every oil is made up of various compounds, sometimes hundreds of compounds that are primarily formed from hydrogen, carbon and oxygen atoms. When oils are high in certain types of compounds, they will share similar characteristics and benefits.

It's not necessary as a beginner to understand the exact chemistry, however hopefully helped you understand how and why there could be so many options for a specific situation. Additionally, because each oil is still different based on the rest of its chemical makeup, how one reacts for one person doesn't mean they will all react that way, or in the same manner for other people. Luckily, there are at least a few or several choices when finding what works best for you.

Latin Names and Chemotypes

Latin Names

Plants (and their oils) have a common name, or an English name, but they also have a botanical name, in Latin, that identifies a particular species.

For example, there are several species of frankincense. The essential oil comes from the gum resins of the trees, typically of these species: *Boswellia Carterii, Boswellia Sacra, and Boswellia Serrata.* Carterii and Sacra are often cause for contentious debate, as some claim that carterii is superior, while others claim that Sacra is better. There are also those who suggest they are actually the same species, just grown in different places, yet the aroma and chemical profiles would indicate they are different. Either way, frankincense is a favorite oil for many and is often noted as being used in the Bible. (In the time of the Bible, Frankincense and Myrhh would not have been in the essential oil form we know them today, as steam distillation had not yet been invented.)

Latin names should always be included on a label. In a few cases, the species difference can mean a difference in therapeutic benefits and safety concerns. For example, you can buy a bottle of lavender, the most common being *Lavandula angustifolia* ((known as true lavender, or English lavender), or it could Spike Lavender, *Lavandula latifolia*. Angustifolia is a very versatile oil with many uses, known to have a wide array of therapeutic benefits. It is one of the safest essential oils available and often known for its calming properties. Latifolia is more stimulating than angustifolia, has a higher content of camphor and should be avoided in pregnancy.

Tip: Officinalis can be seen at times as a second word in a Latin name. This word, in layman's terms, means a plant with medicinal value. It is sometimes used interchangeably for lavender essential oil, "Lavandula Officinalis," instead of Lavandula Angustifolia

Personal examples:

Peppermint essential oil with the Latin name mentha arvensis is actually cornmint. I once purchased a bottle of "organic peppermint" only to find it was not true peppermint. Real peppermint will have the Latin name Mentha Piperita.

Citrus Racemosa and Citrus Paradisi are often used interchangeably for Grapefruit (or Pink Grapefruit.) From what I can determine, name Racemosa is a reference to the fruit itself, whereas paradisi is in regard to the peel, from where the oil is actually obtained. Until recently, as I don't like the fruit, I had never tried Grapefruit essential oil. When I learned of its benefits for weight loss and cellulite I decided to purchase a bottle. Trying to understand if there was a difference between these two Latin names caused me a bit a grief as I wasn't sure which one I needed. From the best I can determine, both are one in the same.

Chemotypes

For certain plants, variants in the environment in which they are grown, including soil, elevation and climate, can result in different chemical constituents. Rosemary, for example, depending on where it's grown, may be botanically identical (and have the same Latin name), but the chemistry of the oil is completely different. In these instances, the differences are noted by chemotype.

Not all plants have chemotypes, but with those that do, it can again mean a difference between benefits and safety uses. For instance, (Rosemary) rosemarinus officinal ct. cineole works well for upper respiratory colds and infections but should be avoided in use with children; ct. camphor can help with fatigue, and ct. verbonene is better than the others for skin care.

Other examples of oils with different chemotypes are Basil and Lemongrass.

Chapter 4: The FDA and USDA

This chapter involves governing agencies in the United States of America. Standards and regulations and bodies that control them will be different in other areas of the world.

FDA Classification

Even though essential oils are used for medicinal and therapeutic purposes, in most cases they are classified as a cosmetic, and are not regulated as drugs by the FDA. This is important for the aromatherapy community and their consumers because getting a product approved as a drug is very involved and very costly, and requires lab and clinical testing. Many who sell essential oils or use them in their various products would not be able to meet the requirements set forth for a drug classification. Under the cosmetics classification those requirements are not necessary.

There is no license or certification required to sell essential oils. An entrepreneur could find a wholesale supplier, come up with a brand name and marketing materials and sell essential oils with no actual knowledge of them. A certified aromatherapist has an education in essential oils, their botanical names, their chemical families, and their safety concerns. They also have to have courses in human physiology/anatomy.

Where it gets tricky is, commercial speech is not fully protected by the First Amendment. With the cosmetic classification, no one, not the new business owner, nor the trained aromatherapist can *sell* essential oils with a claim they can prevent, treat or cure illness or injury.

This can cause a bit of a conundrum as the therapeutic/medicinal value is the primary reason consumers wish to buy them. And, obviously, they need to know which ones to use and how to use them properly. In turn, those selling the oils want to be able to espouse the benefits of using their products. Luckily, the alternative medicine and aromatherapy community had enjoyed a little leniency in promoting the benefits of using essential oils. As a whole, they generally did so responsibly, with proper training and care and encouraging safe use.

There are exceptions though, and those who hold different opinions on what safety requirements are necessary. They may also believe essential oils have greater healing abilities than evidence, even anecdotal evidence can support. People who engage in unproven, exaggerated or false claims have been a growing concern to the industry. These claims could cause harm to the consumers, and cause the entire industry to fall under greater scrutiny.

The latter concern came somewhat to fruition in September of 2014 after sales consultants made claims that their oils could combat Ebola. Although essential oils are being studied for their possible value in preventing and treatment of various diseases, there is no sufficient evidence to support a claim that an essential oil can cure or prevent Ebola.

There were many complaints made to the FDA, resulting in a thorough review and investigation of three different companies, their websites, and even their sales consultants' websites and social media posts. The Food and Drug Administration found many different instances of oils being sold for purposes of treating illness (not limited to Ebola.) Warning letters were sent to the companies with threats that lack of compliance to correct the problems could result in stiff penalties, prosecution and the possibility of their merchandise being seized. These scathing letters are a matter of public record, and can be found on the FDA website, simply by searching key words essential oil. Although many blame "big pharma" for these warnings, it was the result of overzealous marketing and unsubstantiated claims.

The ramifications of this may not yet be fully known, however significant changes are being made of as June 2015. The primary companies involved appear to be taking great measures to ensure they are in compliance and that those who sell the products keep their websites and social media in compliance. Smaller companies and aromatherapists who sell their own line of products are scrambling to ensure they are in compliance as well.

Important to note: The FDA makes no definition of an essential oil in terms of percentages. For instance, there is no rule that states "a bottle only needs to contain 5% of an essential oil for a company to label it as 100% pure." An oil that is "certified pure" or "guaranteed pure" or even "100% pure" has not been tested by any officially recognized, governing body. There *is no* official governing body that tests, certifies or guarantees their quality. A company may have their own process in place for quality control and testing (which sometimes involves hiring an independent third party to test as well) and are guaranteeing or certifying their own standard of quality and purity.

Note: September 2014 was not the first time the FDA sent warning letters. Other, smaller entities had been subject to them in the past. These letters have had greater impact due to the scope and outreach, and large size of the companies who received them.

For further information on how the FDA defines an essential oil and their regulations on labels and ingredients you can visit their page at fda.gov.

USDA – Certified Organic

Just as there is no agency that governs the purity of an essential oil, there is no governing agency that tests oils to determine if they are organic. However, a farm where plants are grown can be certified organic if they meet specified requirements of the United States Department of Agriculture, known as the USDA. It's not an easy process for farmers and growers to obtain certification, so not all oils are from *certified* organic farms. This is not an indication that the oils themselves are not organic, or that they aren't quality oils. Likewise, a certified organic farm doesn't necessarily equate to quality, as there is still no control over what parts of the plant matter was used, how proper the distillation was, and whether or not solvents or adulterations were added.

Chapter 5: Choosing a Brand

Choosing a company you trust can be difficult when getting started. Most of us don't have the ability or knowledge to test essential oils for purity and quality ourselves, so we often have to rely on others to tell us whose oils are the best. There are criteria you can look for in a company though that can aid you in making your decisions.

Tip: You don't ever have to stick with just one brand. Different companies may offer different blends and products you want to try.

Tip: For many consumers, cost matters. The good news is, there are plenty of companies who sell oils at prices that won't be as hard as others on your bank account.

Misleading Labels

There are common phrases on essential oil labels that many frown upon. Phrases such as "certified pure," "aromatherapy grade," or "therapeutic grade." They are considered misleading, and inferring a governing body that again, does not exist. Many go so far as to recommend not purchasing oils from a company who uses any of these terms or phrases on their labels. A rebuttal argument though could be that the labels help differentiate essential oils from other oils (fragrance oils, etc) and adding "therapeutic grade" helps consumers feel confident in their purchases.

Customer Service

When selling products that can influence the health of consumers, proper service to the customers should always be the upmost concern. A vendor should always take measures to ensure quality, understand their products and be able to properly relay the information about them to their consumers.

Personal story: When I first got started, I chose a company based on decent reviews and a good fit for my budget. I was quite pleased with their oils, but at the time, I really knew nothing about them. When I started to take interest in becoming better educated, I went to the company with a few questions. I wanted to know which chemotype of rosemary I had, and I asked why they didn't provide a safety brochure when I purchased oregano, or at least indicate on the bottle that it was a hot oil. Finally, I asked them about wintergreen and if it is safe to use, even though very similar to aspirin. They couldn't answer me on what chemotype their Rosemary was, they were angry I questioned them about a lack of safety materials, and I sent their chemistry based answer (stating erroneously that wintergreen was safe) to a chemist who confirmed the person clearly knew nothing about chemistry or wintergreen. At that point, even though I enjoyed their oils and they actually worked as I wanted them to, I decided it was time to change companies. Since then it has been well established that they were nothing more than "in it for the money." A pretty website and nice labeling didn't make up for the fact that none of the staff had any training on essential oils and the owner had no interest in learning about the products they were selling; that is until the poor customer service, some less than quality independent test results, and many complaints caught up to them over social media. In recent months they have been forced to offer refunds to several unhappy customers and the owner has promised to make significant changes, to learn more about the products sold, and hire an aromatherapist to be on staff.

Here are some things to look for in terms of "customer service" when evaluating companies to purchase from:

1) Do they sell oils known to be rare or difficult to obtain, or are from plants that produce very little oil, for an unrealistically low cost? Essential oils do not have to break the bank for the most part, but there are oils like Melissa, Sandalwood and Rose Otto that are going to be costly. If it seems unrealistically cheap, there's probably a reason. (Exceptions are when a company will pre-dilute an essential oil with a carrier oil. This will lower the cost and is perfectly acceptable as long as they are forthcoming about it.)

2) Do their labels state they are essential oils or do they use other terms such as perfume oil or fragrance oil?

3) Does the company provide safety information for their individual oils that seems to fall within the recommended guidelines of aromatherapists and experts?

4) Do they provide all of the Latin Names and chemotypes (when applicable) for their oils?

5) Do they provide the plant part from which the oil came from?

6) Do they do routine testing on batches of oil (GC/MS) to check for quality and purity? Do they allow consumers to view the reports? (Notice I said routine, and not necessarily every batch. Some smaller businesses can't afford to test every single batch, but this is not an indication the company as a whole is bad.)

7) Do company representatives, customer service/agents seem knowledgeable about the

various oils, their proper use and their
properties?

A company fitting all of this criteria will never be a
guarantee that your oil is pure, however if they show
a care and concern for their customers, and a
knowledge and appreciation for their products, they
are likely taking efforts to ensure quality.

MLMs

In a chapter about choosing a company, I would be
remised if I didn't at least include some information
about multi-level marketing companies. They are a
very hot topic, and the two well known multi-level
marketing companies were recipients of the FDA
letters mentioned in the previous chapter. In social
media discussions they are often referred to as
MLMs.

Multi-level marketing companies have independent
consultants who sell their products, while recruiting
new people to sell. As recruits turn around and
recruit others, chains are formed known as uplines

and downlines. Everyone in the upline benefits from recruits and sales made by the downline. For this reason, products from multi-level marketing companies are typically more expensive. Examples of well known MLM's are Mary Kay and Avon (both cosmetics), and Scentsy (candles).

There are proponents and opponents of MLM's, regardless of the product sold. Opponents don't like the business structure and will often refer to them as a "pyramid scheme," they don't like the cost of the products, feel that consultants (usually women) are asked to impose on friends and family and may end up straining relationships trying to make a sale. Proponents enjoy the freedom to, in a sense, work for yourself, and make extra money based on your own schedule, your own effort, and ability to network and reach out to the community.

The two major MLM's in the essential oil industry are often credited with making aromatherapy more popular and mainstream. As they host parties and classes and introduce friends and family to essential oils, more people are aware of them and are using them than ever before.

Because of the MLMs' global resources, they may have the ability to work hand in hand with their growers and distillers around the world, and may even have their own farms and stills. They can afford regular testing on their products, and given the watchful eye of the community, they can probably meet their claims of purity and excellent quality.

Despite some of the benefits of the MLMs, they are regularly under fire by the aromatherapist community and some consumers. As mentioned they tend to be more expensive, but more importantly, the consultants selling the oils are not required to be certified aromatherapists. They have at times (speaking from personal experience) shared information that is not considered safe, truthful and appropriate by those knowledgeable in the field (as evident by the ebola claims.) Aromatherapists and experts work very hard to reach out to the public and correct some of the wrong information being given, and dispel certain myths that have been perpetuated.

It could be argued however, that the MLM's have also had a fantastic impact on the industry. As mentioned, more people than ever are learning about essential oils and using them. A huge increase in consumers would certainly increase business for others as well, plus has resulted in increased demand for quality among all suppliers.

Personal note: I am in no way affiliated with any essential oil company, MLM or otherwise. In my personal collection of essential oils I have synergies from one of the MLM's that I enjoy, but oils from other companies as well.

Tip: There are many social media groups and websites dedicated to essential oils. If you are going to look to the community for advice on a brand, I encourage you to first seek out groups and websites that have no particular affiliation to any company, who encourage safety, and have aromatherapists and other experts that are on staff or contribute. If you decide an MLM is correct for you, there are plenty of social media groups and websites dedicated to them as well.

Please Note: This section is in no way meant to disparage all independent consultants for MLM's or the actual companies. There are those who care very deeply about safety and encourage proper use, and may have actual aromatherapy certification as well. In addition, consumers and other advocates of essential oils could certainly have a hand in improper recommendations and use. This is simply meant to inform about debates, arguments and discussions that take place regularly in social forums.

Chapter 6: Natural Does Not Mean Safe

Every drop of essential oil is very potent. You may hear comparisons such as 1 drop of lemon essential oil is equal to 75 lemons. A general misconception though is because they are natural, they are safe. This is not true: think poison ivy, poison oak, various forms of wild berries that are known to be poisonous, etc. (There are in fact essential oils available that are considered toxic and aren't typically recommended for use in aromatherapy, including Fig Leaf and Sassafras.) If used safely, however, most essential oils pose very minimal risks.

Many injuries are the result of overuse/overdose and not following general safety guidelines and precautions. This chapter will give an overview of some of those precautions, but it is not meant to replace the advice of an aromatherapist or medical professional. *Please consult with an aromatherapist and your physician when using essential oils, especially if you are pregnant/lactating, elderly, have any serious illnesses/disorders, take prescription medications, and if you plan to use them on or around children and pets.*

Safety Precautions

Possible risks of using essential oils can be skin irritations, allergic reactions, toxicity from overdose or overuse, or they may exacerbate a medical condition. Oils could also be contraindicative to medications one may be taking. Anyone with a history of seizures, asthma, or cancer needs to be aware that there are certain oils that be contraindicative. Always seek the advice of a professional before using any oil.

Example: It's often said that Wintergreen essential oil, which is chemically very much like aspirin, is safe because it is all natural. This is not accurate information, and proper care needs to be taken when using this oil. It should be used only as specifically needed and in very small amounts, it must always be kept away from children, no ingestion and it should never be used on people who can not have aspirin (for instance, those on blood thinners.) These same precautions are true for Birch essential oil as it is very similar to Wintergreen (and aspirin.)

Essential oils should always be diluted when using topically (on skin), and should not be ingested unless under the guidance of an aromatherapist or physician. (Both of these will be covered more extensively later.)

Essential oils should be kept away from the eyes, nose and mouth, and although it's best to wear gloves, at least wash hands thoroughly after working with them. If contact is made with the eyes, flush with saline, or use a vegetable oil to dilute. Seek emergency treatment when necessary.

Personal experience: I learned this one firsthand after working with oregano. I did wash my hands well, and the diluted oil was still so strong that when I rubbed my eye a short time later I was in so much pain I thought I would go blind.

Children

Babies do not have the protective barriers in their skin that adults do. Their skin is much more susceptible to reactions. It is recommended by some to never use essential oils topically on children under the age of 2, and instead to use hydrosols. Others would suggest it is ok to use certain oils such as lavender, Roman and German chamomile if in very low dilutions of only .5 - 1%.

Many essential oils are safe to use around children over the age of 2, including lavender, chamomiles, citrus oils and more. However, they need to be used with proper safety and precaution. Always keep essential oils out of their reach.

NEVER:

> 1) Give a child an oil to drink/ingest. Although it's typically due to entire bottles/large amounts, there have been recorded deaths from children and adults ingesting essential oils. If your child ingests a bottle of essential oil, give them milk, yogurt, or similar product to help dilute and contact poison control and/or emergency services immediately.

2) Put essential oils into the ears (or an adult's), regardless of websites or YouTube videos telling you otherwise.

3) Put an oil in a child's mouth for teething.

4) Use wintergreen or birch on a child, or on an adult who is on a blood thinner or cannot have aspirin.

5) Use rosemary, eucalyptus, peppermint, or other essential oils that contain 1.8 cineole or menthol on younger children under the age of 10. These may open up the airways of an adult, but can have the opposite effect on children, especially infants and toddlers, causing their airways to close and breathing to slow down or become difficult. (Using them in low concentrations in blends with other oils, and diffused throughout a home in small amounts is not likely to cause a reaction, but nonetheless, all parents need to be aware of this danger.)

Pregnancy/Breastfeeding

A woman who is expecting is likely to have much more sensitive skin due to hormone changes. Certain oils need to be used in lower dilutions, especially those that are known skin irritants or phototoxic.

Essential oils are believed capable of passing through the placental barrier and could affect an unborn baby (whether positively or negatively.) They are also able to be passed in very small amounts to babies while nursing. There are oils that may not be recommended for use at all when pregnant or nursing, so please consult with a professional before use.

Skin Reactions

When using essential oils topically (on the skin) they should always be diluted. How to dilute will be discussed in the next chapter, but this section is about *why* dilution is necessary. This completely contradicts mainstream information you may hear from friends or see online, however it is a recommendation that most experts and aromatherapists support and agree with.

There are two main reasons to dilute; the first is toxicity. Although it's not common, too much essential oil could be absorbed through the skin, and over time cause build up in the liver or other areas of the body. The second reason involves various skin reactions. There are typically three different reactions that are possible, and diluting oils makes them less likely to happen: skin irritation, sensitization, and phototoxicity (sometimes referred to as photosensitization.) A popular myth is that a skin reaction to essential oils means your body is detoxing, however experts have dismissed this notion.

Skin Irritation

Certain oils contain known skin (dermal) irritants, or are "hot" oils (if you ever get a drop of oregano on your skin, you'll understand just what that means.) These types of oils, if labeled or marketed appropriately, should always give clear directions that dilution is necessary. . Examples: cinnamon, clove, lemongrass, peppermint, oregano, thyme.

"NEAT" on a label means there are no *known* skin irritants in the oil and can be used without dilution. Unfortunately, this is not considered a safe practice. Remember, we can all react differently, especially those with more sensitive skin such as young children and the elderly. Neat oils should always be diluted properly to reduce any risk of irritation, but even more so, to reduce the risk of sensitization.

Sensitization

Sensitization, in layman's terms, is a type of allergic reaction where the body recognizes something as a foreign invader and reacts to fight it. It does not commonly happen on first use (although it can), as it's typically the result of overuse. A person could have been using an oil regularly for months or even years without issue, when sensitization suddenly occurs. Unlike irritation, this reaction does not just manifest in the area it was applied; it can effect several areas of the body, and may result in a variety of symptoms including nausea, labored breathing and /or need for emergency medical treatment.

Once sensitization has occurred, a person will likely always have a reaction to that oil, and possibly the actual plant in the future. Additionally, it could be merely one component of the oil that caused the reaction, and that component may be found in other oils. Diluting essential oils, and keeping topical use to a minimum can greatly reduce the risk of skin sensitization. Massage therapists are at great risk for sensitization due to their repeated exposure to essential oils. A "NEAT" oil can still lead to skin sensitization.

Tip: Never apply essential oils (neat or diluted) to broken skin. Essential oils in an open wound would increase the chance of sensitization.

Tip: It's best not to use the same oil on your skin for a prolonged period of time. Try rotating oils every week or two to reduce the risk of sensitization.

Phototoxicity

The past few years, news reports have been circulating showing various cases of severe burns after people have worked with citrus fruits in sunlight (often lime.) It's a phenomenon many people aren't even aware of. In short, phototoxicity is a reaction to UV rays that can be brought on by a number of different factors including various diseases, certain skin treatments, pharmaceuticals, and as mentioned, citrus fruits. The result, which can begin to appear quickly or take several hours to fully develop, can be severe burns to the skin.

Certain oils are phototoxic and should be either be avoided in sunlight, or heavily diluted:

Grapefruit and Sweet Myrrh, regardless of how they were obtained.

Lemon, lime, bitter orange and bergamot are phototoxic if they are cold pressed (expressed), instead of steam distilled. These oils commonly *are* cold pressed, so use caution unless you know otherwise from the company providing them.

Tip: You may see phototoxicity referred to as photoirritation or photosensitivity. Phototoxicity is only one type of photosensitivity. Photoallergy is another, but would be very rare with the use of essential oils.

The information provided in this chapter is not necessarily a complete list of precautions or contraindications. Again, please consult with an expert or aromatherapist.

Chapter 7: Methods of Use

There are three common methods of use for therapeutic purposes: inhalation, topical and ingestion. Additional methods that will not be covered in this introductory guide are vaginal and rectal applications (suppositories, enemas.)

Which Method is Best?

Using essential oils on the skin is very popular, but is not always necessary. It's best to consider your purpose for using the oil, and then decide how best to enjoy the benefits.

With topical application, the molecules of essential oils enter the bloodstream, typically in very small amounts, around 5-10% if properly diluted (source: Robert Tisserand). This could be more or less depending on carrier oil/neat application, where it's applied, and other factors. Things that aide in absorption are well hydrated skin, massage and warmth.

Topical use is advantageous in certain situations, such as using oils for cosmetic reasons, or to treat nail fungus, relieve bug bites, and speed the healing of cuts and bruises, etc. Other reasons may be for massaging a localized area afflicted with pain and inflammation.

In contrast, to help with some anxiety, a topical application of a calming oil or blend has not been proven to be any more beneficial than inhaling it. Clinical research supports that by simply inhaling essential oils, the chemical compounds are able to enter the blood stream and pass throughout the body. In fact, there have been suggestions that if topical applications were studied in a controlled environment where subjects were unable to inhale the aromas, the results would potentially show that there are minimal effects if any at all when applying topically for these purposes.

Ingestion is known to be beneficial for certain conditions, whether it be through anecdotal acknowledgement or actual clinical research. For example, peppermint essential oil capsules (available in the supplement section of various pharmacies) are known to help with IBS and other gastrointestinal problems. Essential oils have also shown to be as effective as pharmaceutical antibiotics in certain cases. Unfortunately, (using these same examples), peppermint essential oil could also irritate certain gastrointestinal problems and essential oils may not adequately treat certain or all infections.

Ingestion results in the highest absorption into the body of all three methods, and poses the highest concerns for toxicity and contraindications. For this reason, it is not recommended by most experts/organizations and trained aromatherapists, unless under the appropriate guidance and supervision. This is regardless of the purity / quality of oil. In fact, the higher quality the more potent and thus a greater potential for harm.

Additional Note - It has been suggested that if you have a strong reaction to an oil, and you absolutely love it, this is an indication your spirit and mind are in need of that specific oil. If you have an opposite reaction and absolutely hate the odor, this indicates you need the oil to help you detox. Your reaction is because it has already started working on the toxins that are built up in your body. This suggestion has been debunked by experts.

Tip: A common recommendation is to put oils on the bottom of the feet, but this has been somewhat debunked by many. The bottoms of the feet are too tough, and the numerous sweat glands prevent much, if any at all, from entering your body. There are really only two valid reasons for applying this way: 1) You are treating an issue on the feet or 2) You want to use the oil topically, but want a less sensitive area of skin. Any other reason is unnecessary as the primary benefit you will be receiving from applying them to the feet is the aroma you're smelling. The effect would be the same if you applied it elsewhere (such as wrists, neck, etc.)

Tip: There is no evidence to support that essential oils will have any greater effect when using them on reflexology points.

Inhalation

Methods of inhalation include:

1) Simply opening a bottle and breathing in the aroma. Not necessarily the best option, as you may want to do this several times a day. Every time you open the bottle you are exposing the entire bottle to more oxygen which will shorten the shelf life.

2) Using an inhaler. – Inhalers can be purchased online and in some natural stores. Often times they take a similar shape to a tampon, so some vendors have made attempts to give them a more appealing design, such as like a tube of lipstick. To use an inhaler you simply place at the bottom of or just inside each nostril and breathe in the aroma.

3) Diffusers – There are a variety of options for diffusing, including reed diffusers, electric cool mist or heat diffusers, atomizers/nebulizers

designed for essential oils, candle diffusers and fan diffusers. There are also diffusers that you can plug into your car for drives and road trips.

4) Steam / steam tent. This is boiling water, and adding a few drops of oil and breathing in the steam. Many people will do a steam tent – this is where you make a "tent" over yourself and the steaming pot/bowl/cup. You can also leave out the "tent" part if it's too strong for you, as it is a very quick and rapid absorption and is not the gentlest method. It is more effective than diffusing. Keep your eyes closed during steam inhalation to help avoid irritation.

5) On a cotton square or tissue, etc. When you can't diffuse and are on the go, you can keep cotton or tissue saturated with a few drops and pull it out as needed. I will often keep mine in a little sealed plastic bag in my pocket. You can also place a cotton pad near your pillow at night.

6) A couple of drops on a shirt collar. This is a method I use for my pre-school aged child with

lemon essential oil, to help slow down a runny nose. I would do this for her for the couple of hours she was in school. I have never noticed the oils leaving stains on her collar but they may, so I don't necessarily recommend this for finer outfits.

7) Humidifier – some will use essential oils in their humidifier, however, caution is needed as it could harm your unit.

8) Jewelry – There is jewelry that you can buy that works as a

Diffusing or breathing in the aromas in high concentrations should be done in intervals, for instance, 15 minutes on, 30 minutes off. Constant exposure to highly concentrated vapors is not recommended. A couple of drops in a diffuser in a large room is safe, but several drops in a powerful nebulizer, especially in a smaller, not well ventilated room could be more harmful than beneficial. There are diffusers you can purchase that allow you to set these timed intervals.

Topical

Methods of topical use can include:

1) Full body massages – calming oils would likely be chosen, as well as those that are beneficial to the skin

2) Spot treatments (acne, bruises, skin tags, etc.)

3) For use as a perfume

4) On specific areas to help with muscle cramps, joint pain, etc.

5) Bathtub (This ends up being topical and inhalation.) Because oils in a bath will still come in contact with the skin and possibly mucous membranes, oils should be diluted and then use a dispersing agent (such as bath salts.)

Ingesting

Never ingest essential oils without the aid of an expert.

Ingesting should not be done for preventative measures, and instead (again, under the guide of a professional) for specific treatment purposes.

Essential oils do not mix in water and, despite the popularity of this, should not be added to drinking water.

If you have discussed ingestion with a professional and have concluded it's appropriate for you, it's best to use a gel cap, or other soluble medium to reduce any risks. There are also edible dispersants that you can add to water to help with diluting and mixing.

GRAS (Generally regarded as safe) as designated by the FDA for certain essential oils is mistakenly used as a suggestion that essential oils can be ingested without concern. GRAS is pertaining to food additives. Although a drop of oregano essential oil may add some spice to your spaghetti, when putting a drop in your favorite pasta sauce it is dispersed among all of the other ingredients and then mixed in with the pasta as well. This is vastly different from putting a drop of oregano in your mouth to swallow, or in a cup of water and drinking it.

A common misconception is that in France, essential oils are regularly ingested in everyday life. The French do incorporate ingesting as part of their use of essential oils, but typically under the care of medical professionals, and possibly in combination with conventional medicines.

Tip: Ingesting is different than using an essential oil as part of an oral care routine for your teeth and gums. Oil pulling (with coconut oil, or other vegetable oils), an old method of oral care, has sprung into popularity, and a very low dilution with an essential oil such as peppermint or spearmint would in general be considered a safe practice. In addition, many people are making their own toothpastes with an essential oil as part of their ingredients. As it is being spit out, it is not considered ingesting.

Never use clove essential oil for a baby who is teething. This is a hot oil, can burn their mouths and is very unpleasant to taste. In adults it has been well recorded as a time old treatment for dental pain and use, and is widely used today, but serious side effects can occur with misuse or overuse. These side effects include nausea, seizures, burns, and liver or kidney failure.

Tip: Essential oils do not contain vitamins or nutrients. This is a popular myth, but any vitamins or nutrients that could have found their way to the oils would be destroyed when obtaining the oils.

Chapter 8: Carriers, Diluting and Blending

As discussed in the previous chapter, essential oils should be diluted before applying to your skin. To dilute, aromatherapists and consumers use carrier oils.

Fixed / Carrier Oils

Unlike essential oils, fixed oils are *nonvolatile* oils from plants or animals. Although there are exceptions, most are vegetable oils, and many are derived from various seeds and nuts. They can be obtained using the preferred method of cold press expression, or can also be steamed or solvent extracted. When used in soaps and lotions they are referred to as base oils or fixed oils, but for purposes of essential oils, they are typically referred to as a carrier oil.

A somewhat popular myth is that carrier oils "carry" an essential oil into the skin. Fixed oils have large molecules that are unable to penetrate through the skin. For this reason, using a carrier oil will result in less absorption, and the rate of absorption can vary depending on the carrier chosen. However, if you apply an essential oil <u>NEAT</u> (undiluted, straight on to your skin) without a carrier, the oil will evaporate more quickly, also reducing the amount of oil actually absorbed into your body. A carrier oil slows down the evaporation rate.

There are a number of different carrier oils to choose from, and all have different properties and benefits of their own as well as various shelf lives. Some common, popular choices for carrier oils are Sweet Almond Oil (People with nut allergies should avoid use), Fractionated Coconut Oil, Coconut Oil (solid at room temperature), Grape Seed Oil and Jojoba Oil. Olive oil can be used, however due to the aroma and thickness isn't always a popular choice.

Other Carriers

Carriers can also include lotions, butters (such as cocoa butter), witch hazel and more. Many lotions can already contain their own blends of essential oils and fragrances so be sure to check the ingredients. Avoid using baby oil and any moisturizers that contain mineral oil, as well as petroleum jelly. These can prevent absorption of the essential oils as well as clog pores in the skin.

Dilution Recommendations

As a general guideline, for daily topical use a 2% dilution for <u>most oils</u> is considered safe. For short term use, 3% up to 10% could be appropriate, and there may be instances where up to a 25% dilution or higher for spot application treatments may be recommended by trained aromatherapists.

Exceptions to the 2% guideline would be for topical use on the elderly, pregnant women and children, where the recommendations are between .5 – 1% dilution. Additionally, certain oils that have known skin irritants or are hot oils require heavier dilution. Common examples are lemongrass, wintergreen, oregano, peppermint, thyme and other hot oils, as well as phototoxic oils that will be exposed to sunlight. Always check the label and instructions for your specific oil, refer to the company you are purchasing from and when necessary due to age or health concerns, consult with an aromatherapist or other trained professional.

When oils are properly diluted, and being used topically for a specific purpose, you can generally apply them regularly, as needed. (As with everything there are exceptions though, such as Wintergreen and Birch, which need used sparingly.)

How to Dilute and Measure

To dilute an essential oil, simply mix it with your chosen carrier. You can pre-mix and store, using glass containers, or do spot applications when needed.

Diluting per teaspoon:

1 Drop of an essential oil in 1 teaspoon of carrier = 1% dilution, 2 drops = 2%, 3 drops =3% and so on.

Diluting per ounce:

6 drops of an essential oil per 1 ounce of carrier = 1% dilution, 12 drops = 2% and so on.

Diluting per Milliliters (ML):

1 Drop of essential oil to 5ML of carrier = 1%, 2 Drops to 10ML = 2% and so on.

Tip: There are 5 ML in one teaspoon, almost 15 ML in one tablespoon and 30 ML in one ounce.

Blending Essential Oils

There are many wonderful blends, commonly known as synergies, on the market. They are usually very strategically formulated by experts based on plant chemicals and properties, for therapeutic reasons, and/or aromas for fragrance or perfumery. Synergies are often labeled in such a way to make you aware of their intended benefits. For example, an anti-anxiety blend could be named something like Comfort Blend, or Anxiety Be Gone Blend.   Always check the list of ingredients in the blend.

Although synergies *can* be a very complicated science, you can also have fun making blends at home as well.

To create blends for fragrance purposes, one would want to have a nice blend of oils that includes top notes, middle notes, and base notes. A top note will evaporate the quickest – these typically have more of a fruity scent. The middle notes are more of a floral fragrance, and the base notes, which are more viscous and have a slower evaporation time, tend to be a deeper, woodsier, earthy scent. I have not included a list of the various oils and their note classification for this beginner's guide, but this information is readily available from multiple sites online.

Tip: When making a perfume with essential oils for the first time, choose a carrier that has a neutral odor. Then, add your base notes first, this is the aroma that will last the longest, then add middle notes, and then top notes.

When creating blends for therapeutic purposes, the notes don't need to be considered, rather just their therapeutic properties. For example, for an anti-inflammatory blend you could look to add various oils such as eucalyptus, peppermint, myrrh, ginger, helichrysum and roman chamomile. Once you have chosen your oils based on your need, then you can make additions if necessary if it's not appealing in terms of fragrance. Remember every drop used in the blend needs an appropriate amount of carrier oil added to it (if the blend will be used topically.)

Tip: When creating blends for a therapeutic purpose, it is always best to allow them at least a couple of days or more (up to a week) to mix. I have noticed a big difference between using my own inflammation blend on day 1 versus day 7. (Important to note for perfume blends, the aroma will be different as well.)

Tip: When making blends, even if just experimenting, always take careful notes of what oils you used and how much.

Tip: The order of how you add oils to your blend will not change the chemical properties or the aroma of the oils. Those changes only occur with time.

Chapter 9: Storage and Accessories

Shelf Life and Storage

It's very exciting when you buy essential oils, or order them and have them delivered to your door. The urge to open them all up and try them all out is normal and perfectly fine. One thing to keep in mind though is every time oil is exposed to oxygen, it's shortening the shelf life.

Shelf life varies for certain oils, depending on the oil's chemistry / chemical families. There is no actual expiration date as that can vary greatly due to exposure to oxygen and the way it's stored. However, for a general beginning guideline, citrus oils are only good for about a year, other oils can last 3-4 years, while the more viscous oils can last for several, 6-10, years.

The best place for essential oils is in the refrigerator or freezer. If not refrigerated, the next best place is dark, cool areas. Don't leave bottles of essential oils sitting on your window sill. They don't do well with heat or light (natural or artificial). When working with essential oils, transferring them to other containers, etc, remember, the more air space available in the container, the more oxygen they are exposed to. Always use glass containers.

ALWAYS store essential oils away from the reach of children.

Tip: Mixing an essential oil (or carrier oil) with fractionated coconut oil can extend its shelf life.

Accessories

First, remember it's best to use gloves when working with essential oils. Second, when you are experimenting, dividing oils for friends and family, or making blends for specific purposes make sure you label everything. Here is a small list of accessories you can find to aid you in using and creating with essential oils:

Roller bottles – these have a little roller ball on the end for quick and easy application. Make a small blend, or dilute your favorite essential oil with a carrier and place in bottle. Snap the roller back in and you already have a pre-diluted mix to carry and roll on when necessary.

Amber glass bottles – These can be purchased with or without droppers. They are dark in color for proper storage.

Plastic transfer pipettes. - These are great for quick transfer of drops of oil and controlling the amount desired. Can allow for more precision than opening an essential oil bottle and hoping the right number of drops come out.

1 ML Amber Glass Vials. - These tiny vials can be great for use as samples, if you are sharing them with friends or family. Can also be used if your main oil bottles start getting too much air space and you want to transfer them to something smaller to reduce the oxygen exposure.

Cap Stickers – If you store all of your essential oils together and upright, and have several of them, trying dig through all of them to find the oil you are looking for gets a little annoying if they don't have cap labels.

Some companies offer them on their bottles, others do not. Luckily you can purchase them, very cheap, made specific to the size of a typical essential oil cap. Often times they come pre-printed, so you can just peel and stick. In addition to the pre-printed you will also often get several that are blank so you can fill in your own label for your different blends.

Spray caps – great to use for linen sprays, making your own fragrance, etc.

Conclusion

Thank you for taking the time to read this book, I hope you have found it very helpful as you consider making essential oils a part of your life. They can be a wonderful, natural alternative for you and your family once you know how to use them safely. Remember to always consult with an aromatherapist if you have serious medical conditions, you are considering ingesting essential oils, or if you are pregnant/nursing. Don't discount safety advice, such as keeping oils away from eyes, washing hands thoroughly after using, and storing them safely away from children. Avoid overuse, and always dilute for topical application. Seek out companies whom are dedicated to their oils and their uses, and take responsibility for the wellbeing of their customers by providing any pertinent information. Following these guidelines will get you on the right path to enjoying the benefits of essential oils.

www.ingramcontent.com/pod-product-compliance
Lightning Source LLC
Chambersburg PA
CBHW071227280526
45787CB00002B/837